I0691716

CONTENTS

1   Having a healthy, mind, body and soul

To discover the ultimate path to well being, you have to reach inside of your mind, body and soul like you never have before. This takes a conscious effort or *massive action* as Anthony Robbins most aptly calls it. Anthony Robbins who is probably regarded as the greatest motivational speaker on the planet says that you need to take *massive action* in his book Unlimited Power (Published by Simon & Schuster 1989). In the last 10 years I have read several hundred self-help books and regard Unlimited Power as the listened to him for many an hour.

Anthony Robbins is exactly right. There is no point in procrastinating on doing something. You have to actually do it. You have to look inside of yourself and ask who you are as a human being and what you are capable of. Then do it.

Once you discover who you are you can then discover what you want and then start doing it. It really is as simple as that and not rocket science just life.

During this book I have decided to split the journey to Ultimate Well Being into eight manageable steps (It's like two Stephen Covey books in one – only joking, Steve I am a big fan of your books… Please keep writing). Whilst you go through each step and you are also taking a step forward and are therefore a step closer to Ultimate Well Being. Each step will take you that little bit closer to 100% mental well being. See this book as an examination of yourself. You will be able to pass but you will have to challenge yourself to progress. This book is an opportunity for you to test yourself and give yourself 100% success as you are the examiner of your life. Nobody else is responsible for how you feel... Just you... That is the reality. See this examination as a confirmation that you and anyone can choose to be a success and even rid yourself of your ego in the process so you can lead a more fulfilled life and have a more positive impact on the world. I repeat. You are boils down to you and not anybody else.

This is not just another self help book. Even if it was I do not think that would necessarily be a bad thing. I like self help books. They fill your head with positive things and day to day people can easily be bombarded with more negative than positive thoughts so a self-help can reprogramme positivism. My first two books document how I lived a life of manic depression and cured myself. (If you feel this is dubious please break your pattern, open your mind, change your belief system do whatever it takes to accept this as fact and then read on!) I have been in the depths of despair and welcomed positivism and enlightenment into my life and made the permanent switch autobiographical memoirs from people who suffer 'mental illness' as I have changed my life and I am not using some kind of theoretical system like most other self help books where the personal suffering or the author and their biographical/autobiographical history and weaknesses are a mystery. Reading this book is a unique opportunity for you to totally enhance your life and reach new standards in every aspect of your life so you can be totally empowered.

You will be able to be a *novus homo* as they say in Latin. A new man as the amazing Roman orator Cicero was in 63BC when he became a member of the Equestrian Order through his achievements instead of hard to identify with the life of someone over 2000 years ago in another city then think of rap.

Think of Eminem's lyrics in the film 8 Mile. The Director of 8 Mile said that writing the lyrics for 8 Mile made Eminem go deeper inside himself than at any other time in his life. As Eminem says in the most famous track he wrote for the movie "*If you had one chance, one opportunity in life… would you capture it or let it slip*". The implication is that you capture it and this is exactly what Eminem does in the film 8 Mile and exactly why he won the contest and went back to work to save up for his studio time so Rabbit would become a famous rapper just like Eminem is.

Would you capture it or let it

opportunity came along for me to make a rap album I managed to capture it and not let it slip. I have recently launched this rap album. Although it was a very steep learning curve over a short period of time and a lot of hard work it was much easier than I thought. The album is called "A Can of Madness", the same name of my book and autobiography on living with manic depression published in 2002 by Chipmunkapublishing. I had once chance to do a rap album and took it. It all started when a volunteer in the Chipmunka office called Ama was reading the rap I wrote in "A Can of Madness" and said that she liked it and that she had a friend whose boyfriend was a rapper. I've always loved hip-hop ever since I racism globally. I liked writing lyrics but never really thought of doing an album or performing. Soon enough I met Ama's friend and the rapper. His name was Ryan and at 17 years of age he had his own label Raskil Records. I was amazed how good the rappers were on his label, especially as most of them were teenagers and they wanted to help people with mental illness so within 6 weeks I had paid for and organised two rap events for them to perform for the very first time live. At the first event one of my friends came along whose rap name is Howling. He was 23 years of age at the time and multi-talented and introduced me to his friend Avarice who made his beats. Avarice happens to be a brilliant producer, lyricist and rapping in time to the beats to the lyrics that I had written a few years earlier. This consisted of several evening sessions after work in Chipmunka's main offices in central London. Then we spent one day round his house as he has his own studio and within four months of meeting him I had launched my rap album.

I mention this as an example to you that not only like Eminem you can do anything like making a rap album if you wanted to. It's just a little example of how if you have a good feeling for something that you should just go for it and reap the rewards whether they are emotional, financial, psychological or spiritual. In return I wanted to help Avarice so kept in touch and I am helping to promote his talented rappers in British Hip Hop.

Moment of Decision

As Anthony Robbins tells us it is in the moment of our decision when our lives change or make a *paradigm shift* as Stephen Covey calls it. Anyone who hears and connects with Eminem in the film 8 Mile could think of something in their lives that they have been hesitant about and would choose to go for it. If you read this book with this positive mentality and decisiveness then you will achieve Ultimate Well Being. So congratulations to you dear reader for taking that quantum leap (Yes VISUALISE IT RIGHT NOW... feel good... that's not good enough.... feel great... feel

We get what we focus on in life. In order to have a healthy mind, body and soul you need to treat these conditions as achievable qualities. Everyone has them so if you don't feel it stop moping around and just zap yourself with some amazing, fantastic, energising sense of feeling great for yourself, other people and the world as a whole. If someone tells you that you have manic depression and a chemical imbalance in the brain, they do not know what they are talking about. You can alter your chemistry by getting more oxygen and jogging in the morning. No psychiatrist has ever proven that there is something wrong with your brain so snap out of believing it. Life is worth living. Take it from me I know I have been it and then watch the last 5 minutes again. feel the sensation of turning your life around. It really is that is easy. If Forest Gump can achieve the impossible then so can you my dear friend. And if you can... so can anyone...

So let's deconstruct having a healthy mind, body and soul into three parts. First let's break them down into three separate parts. Then we will show how they are all connected.

Having a healthy mind.

Having a healthy mind is as achievable as you want it to be. Let's set some targets. Say out loud "my goal is to have a healthy mind body and soul 24 hours a day seven days a week for the rest of my life." Feel good? Well mind. Then out loud. Now try doing something fun with your body, like smiling, while you are doing this or even be more adventurous and try a flying kick... something to give you more oxygen and change your physiology so you are in a PEAK state....... Repeat this three times... Feeling Great..... Now CONTINUE.

Those of you who have been to an Anthony Robbins Seminar will know exactly what I am talking about. Don't worry if you haven't. Ever seen Paul McKenna? Now you have re-programmed your mind as Paul McKenna would say to make this feeling of feeling GREAT a reality. The more intensely you practice this INCANTATION and awaken the more real it will become. Why not commit to chanting to your first step to Ultimate Well Being three times a yourself and give yourself 1% towards Ultimate Well Being.

Congratulations, you only have 99% to go. This will be as easy as you wish it to be. And you will remember the decisions you have made in this book forever because you are consciously choosing to do so. Now celebrate as if your favourite football team has just scored! Or for all you ladies reading this as if you have just bought a beautiful outfit that you feel stunning in and the man or woman of your dreams walks straight up to you and asks you out. LOL... Or something else that will give you the same amazing feeling. Having just met your loved one for the first time! An end to world poverty... Every religion becoming friends... Something totally awesome and loving so you will NEVER FORGET THIS BEAUTIFUL MOMENT. Do

Close your eyes and have some beautiful intensity and love that will improve your life and the lives of those you love and even those that you haven't met forever. Feel the love and relax in a state of being.

Congratulations you are now fully on your way to ACHIEVING 100% and ULTIMATE WELL BEING, What's remarkable too is that this is a gift that you can pass on both consciously and unconsciously. You can pass this on so you can help other people and the world as one. Eckhart Tolle writes about this in The Power of Now. He is an amazing person. For the first 29 years of his life he was severely mentally ill. Then a profound spiritual transformation virtually dissolved his old identity and radically changed the course of his life. He did not know who he was but spent three years on writes in his introduction of the Power of Now that he lived in a state of almost continuous anxiety interspersed with periods of suicidal depression. One night he woke up with absolute dread that was so intense, more intense than he had ever experienced. He had a deep loathing for everything in the world his misery was compounded as he loathed himself more than anything else. During his moment of the deepest psychological pain that he ever experienced he broke through in to a higher state of consciousness. Tolle writes:

"I cannot live with myself any longer." This was the thought that kept repeating itself in my mind. Then suddenly I became aware of what a peculiar thought it was. "Am I one or two? If I cannot live with myself, there must be two of me: the 'I' and the 'self' that 'I'

His massive action, paradigm step, step into Ultimate Well Being, step into being, personal transformation or whatever you want to call it, shows that anything is possible for a human being. Tolle is a living example that anyone's life no matter how desperate can improve.

The same is true of any kind of mental illness including manic depression. I know this because I achieved the transition myself. When I was 17 I was diagnosed with manic depression. From the ages 17-25 I spent over 1 year of my life in five different psychiatric hospitals. By the age of 29 I had made a 90% recovery but was still part of the medical system. In September 2005 I made a life changing decision after meeting Robbins who work I'd been following and using as one of my techniques for inspiration in life

manifested and that I would come off the medication that was poisoning my mind and to come off it forever. I also managed to get sponsored by the NHS to go to his events so that was a bonus and felt justified in receiving this gift as my day job is a social entrepreneur and learning his techniques would enable me to help more people anyway. Robbins and his techniques had helped but without being a social entrepreneur I would never had been able to make a full recovery. Both positive outcomes could be maximised to help even more people and give myself more personal growth and happiness.